--- WELCOME ---

The Healing Rebel, Nourished By Nature Recipes & Journal

Recipes

For more amazing recipes
Find Janice www.blognourishedbynature.com

RECIPE CARD

Falafel Bites

These wee falafel bites tick all the boxes and are ideal for a quick and healthy lunch. They are super easy, don't involve any faffing around with hot oil and a frying pan and are packed full of flavour and nutrition. They are literally fat free and gluten free.

Delicious served warm in a wrap with hummus and salad or just on their own as a snack!
Makes 12 small falafel

INGREDIENTS

- 1 TIN CHICKPEAS, RINSED & WELL DRAINED
- 1 MEDIUM CARROT, GRATED
- 1 SMALL RED ONION, GRATED OR FINELY CHOPPED
- 1 TABLESPOON TAHINI
- 1 TEASPOON PAPRIKA
- 1 TEASPOON GROUND CUMIN
- 1 TEASPOON GROUND TURMERIC
- 1 TEASPOON GROUND CORIANDER
- 1 CLOVE OF GARLIC, CRUSHED OR ¼ TEASPOON GARLIC POWDER
- 1 TEASPOON SEA SALT
- FRESHLY GROUND BLACK PEPPER
- SESAME SEEDS (OPTIONAL)

METHOD

1. QUITE SIMPLY PUT THE DRAINED CHICKPEAS, GRATED CARROT, RED ONION AND THE SPICES AND SEA SALT IN A BOWL AND ROUGHLY BLEND WITH A HAND BLENDER OR JUST USE A POTATO MASHER.
2. ADD THE TAHINI AND MIX TOGETHER.
3. IF THE MIXTURE IS TOO WET, YOU CAN ADD MORE CHICKPEAS, MORE GRATED CARROT OR A TABLESPOON OF POLENTA. YOU WANT THE MIXTURE TO HOLD TOGETHER.
4. LIGHTLY GREASE A BAKING TRAY, WET YOUR HANDS, TAKE SPOONFULS OF THE MIXTURE AND SHAPE INTO BALLS. PUT THEM ON THE TRAY. FLATTEN THEM SLIGHTLY. MAKES ABOUT 12 SMALL FALAFEL. YOU CAN ROLL THEM IN SESAME SEEDS BEFORE YOU BAKE THEM, FOR A WEE BIT OF ADDED TEXTURE IF YOU LIKE!
5. BAKE IN THE OVEN AT 180C FOR AROUND 20 TO 25 MINUTES, TURNING HALFWAY THROUGH COOKING, UNTIL THEY ARE NICELY BROWNED.
6. SERVE AND ENJOY!

NOTES

RECIPE CARD

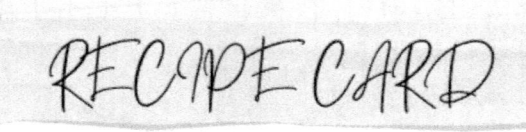

Puff Pastry Rolls

Now we all know that puff pastry isn't very healthy and even less so when filled with a greasy assortment of dodgy ingredients so my delicious gut healthy version is harnessing all the prebiotic power of leeks, red onions, spinach, garlic, courgette and chickpeas with great flavour and polyphenols with lemon zest, flat leaf parsley and thyme from the garden.

These are equally good eaten cold for a picnic lunch.

INGREDIENTS

- 1 PACK OF READY MADE PUFF PASTRY
- 2 TO 3 MEDIUM LEEKS, WASHED, HALVED LENGTHWAYS AND SLICED
- 1 TABLESPOON RAPESEED OR OLIVE OIL
- 1 MEDIUM RED OR WHITE ONION, FINELY SLICED
- 2 CLOVES GARLIC, CRUSHED OR FINELY CHOPPED
- 1/2 BAG OF BABY LEAF SPINACH
- 1 COURGETTE, GRATED
- 1 TIN CHICKPEAS, DRAINED
- 100G VEGAN FETA, CUT INTO SMALL CUBES (OPTIONAL)
- ZEST OF 1 LEMON
- 2 TABLESPOONS FRESH HERBS, FLAT LEAF PARSLEY, SAGE, OREGANO, THYME OR ROSEMARY
- COUPLE TABLESPOONS PLANT MILK
- 1 TSP LINSEEDS, 1TSP CHIA SEEDS, 1 TSP SESAME SEEDS
-

NOTES

METHOD

1. HEAT A TABLESPOON OF RAPESEED OIL IN A LARGE PAN, WITH A PINCH OF SALT, ADD THE LEEKS AND ONIONS AND COOK GENTLY FOR 10 MINUTES UNTIL SOFT AND SWEET.
2. ADD THE GRATED COURGETTE, GARLIC, SPINACH AND COOK FOR ANOTHER 5 MINUTES OR SO THEN ADD THE DRAINED CHICKPEAS.
3. IF YOUR MIXTURE IS WET THEN DRAIN ANY EXCESS LIQUID, THEN TRANSFER TO A LARGE BOWL.
4. ADD THE CHOPPED HERBS, LEMON ZEST AND SOME SEA SALT AND BLACK PEPPER.
5. ADD THE CUBED FETA, IF USING.
6. LEAVE THE FILLING ASIDE TO COOL
7. HEAT THE OVEN TO 220C
8. UNROLL THE PUFF PASTRY ONTO A FLOURED SURFACE, THEN CUT IN HALF LENGTHWAYS SO YOU HAVE 2 LONG THIN RECTANGLES.
9. IF YOU ARE USING A BLOCK OF PUFF PASTRY, THEN YOU WILL HAVE TO ROLL IT OUT INTO A THIN RECTANGLE, THEN CUT IT INTO 2.
10. WITH THE LONG SIDE TOWARD YOU, SPOON HALF YOUR FILLING MIXTURE ALONG THE MIDDLE OF THE RECTANGLE, SHAPING IT INTO A SAUSAGE SHAPE WITH YOUR HANDS.
11. BRUSH THE FAR AWAY EDGE OF THE PASTRY WITH SOME PLANT MILK.
12. PULL THE NEAR SIDE OF THE PASTRY OVER THE FILLING, THEN CAREFULLY PULL THE MILK WASHED SIDE ON TOP AND PRESS IT TO SEAL.
13. CAREFULLY TURN THE WHOLE THING OVER SO THE JOIN IS AT THE BOTTOM, THEN CUT THE ROLL INTO 6 OR 8 EQUAL PIECES.
14. REPEAT WITH THE OTHER RECTANGLE.
15. PUT THE ROLLS ONTO A LIGHTLY GREASED BAKING TRAY, BRUSH WITH PLANT MILK AND SPRINKLE WITH THE SEED MIX.
16. BAKE FOR 20 TO 25 MINUTES UNTIL GOLDEN BROWN AND CRISPY.
17. YOU MAY HAVE TO TURN THE TRAY HALFWAY THROUGH FOR EVEN BAKING, IF YOUR OVEN HAS A HOTSPOT.

RECIPE CARD

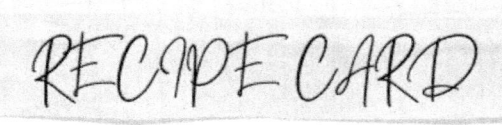

Tabbouleh

Tabbouleh is a delicious Middle Eastern salad dish, made with bulgur wheat but you can substitute quinoa as a gluten free alternative. Chickpeas, goat's cheese, feta cheese, sun-dried tomatoes, olives, avocado and chopped peppers are all great additions for extra diversity points.

Feel free to use any combination of herbs, flat leaf parsley, basil, coriander and mint are all good, the more the better!

INGREDIENTS

- 1 RED ONION, FINELY CHOPPED
- SMALL BUNCH OF SPRING ONIONS CHOPPED
- JUICE OF 1 LEMON
- 2 HANDFULS OF CORIANDER OR FLAT LEAF PARSLEY, CHOPPED
- 2 HANDFULS OF MINT, CHOPPED
- 1 CUP OF BULGUR WHEAT
- ½ CUCUMBER DICED
- 10 CHERRY TOMATOES, HALVED
- 2 TABLESPOONS EXTRA VIRGIN OLIVE OIL, FLAXSEED OIL OR RAPE-SEED OIL
- HIMALAYAN SEA SALT TO TASTE

METHOD

1. PLACE BULGUR WHEAT IN A BOWL, COVER WITH 2 CUPS BOILING WATER AND LEAVE TO SIT FOR 30 MINUTES
2. CHOP THE RED ONION, SPRING ONIONS, TOMATOES AND HERBS
3. CUT THE CUCUMBER IN HALF LENGTHWAYS, SCOOP OUT THE SEEDS AND CHOP INTO SMALL CHUNKS
4. DRAIN THE BULGUR THROUGH A SIEVE TO GET RID OF EXCESS WATER THEN USE A FORK TO SEPARATE THE GRAINS. PUT IT INTO YOUR BEST LOVELY SALAD BOWL. ADD CHOPPED VEGETABLES, HERBS, LEMON JUICE, OLIVE OIL AND SALT TO SEASON
5. LIGHTLY TOASTED PUMPKIN/SUNFLOWER SEEDS, CHOPPED NUTS, FETA CHEESE CUBES CAN ALL BE ADDED TO ADD EXTRA PROTEIN, GOOD FATS AND A BIT OF TEXTURE!
6. LEAVE TABBOULEH IN THE FRIDGE FOR A FEW HOURS BEFORE SERVING TO ALLOW FULL FLAVOURS TO DEVELOP.

NOTES

RECIPE CARD

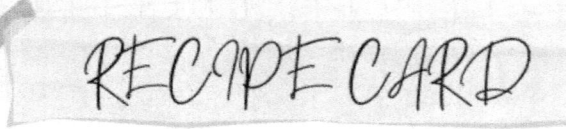

Probiotic Potato Salad

A supercharged version of a summer classic! This is a really delicious and versatile recipe, which is perfect for summer BBQ's and al fresco dining. There isn't really an exact recipe, you simply cook your potatoes then add any extras you fancy!

Cold potatoes are high in resistant starch, a great food source for our gut bacteria.

INGREDIENTS

USE NEW POTATOES OR SMALL SALAD POTATOES, SIMPLY COOK THEM IN SALTED WATER, UNTIL COOKED BUT STILL FIRM, DRAIN AND COOL.

ALL SORTS OF PREBIOTIC FIBRE CAN BE ADDED TO UP THE HEALTH BENEFITS; SOME GREAT OPTIONS:

- SLICED RED ONION, SPRING ONION OR CHIVES, FOR ONIONY FLAVOUR
- GHERKINS, CAPERS, OLIVES, RADISH BOMBS OR SLICED RADISHES, FOR TANG
- FRESH LEAFY HERBS, MINT, FENNEL, DILL, BASIL, LOVAGE, FLAT-LEAF PARSLEY FOR POLYPHENOLS

A CREAMY DRESSING MADE FROM EQUAL AMOUNTS (AROUND ¼ CUP OF EACH) OF

- MAYONNAISE VEGAN OR NORMAL
- PLAIN GREEK OR NATURAL YOGHURT (VEGAN IF YOU WANT)
- A COUPLE OF TABLESPOONS OF SPICY RADISH BOMB BRINE. ADD A TSP OF MUSTARD AND/OR GARLIC POWDER IF YOU DON'T HAVE RADISH BRINE.

METHOD

SIMPLY MIX THE DRESSING INGREDIENTS TOGETHER, AND ADJUST THE SEASONING TO TASTE. GREEK YOGHURT MAKES A REALLY THICK AND CREAMY DRESSING OR A VEGAN ALTERNATIVE PLAIN YOGHURT; THIS ADDS MORE PROBIOTICS TO THE PLATE! POUR THE DRESSING OVER THE COOLED POTATOES AND YOUR CHOSEN EXTRA INGREDIENTS AND IT'S READY!

- TO MAKE THIS MORE OF A MEAL YOU CAN ADD CHICKPEAS, BLANCHED GREEN BEANS, COLD BOILED EGGS OR AVOCADO.
- FOR A BIT OF CRUNCH ADD SOME DRY TOASTED PUMPKIN OR SUNFLOWER SEEDS

NOTES

RECIPE CARD

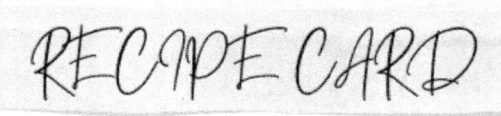

Wild rice salad

This is a beautiful salad, high in diversity points and flavour. Cold rice is high in resistant starch, and all the veggies are prebiotic too so this is a real treat for our gut microbes.
Capers, olives, edible flowers, or any ferments can be added for additional points!

Serves 4 - 6

INGREDIENTS

- 250G WILD RICE, BLACK RICE, RED RICE OR BROWN RICE
- 1 CARROT, GRATED
- 5 OR 6 LEAVES OF CURLY KALE, CUT FROM THE STEMS AND FINELY SLICED
- 3 TABLESPOONS RAISINS, SOAKED FOR AN HOUR AND ROUGHLY CHOPPED
- 6 RADISHES, TRIMMED AND FINELY DICED
- 6 SUN DRIED TOMATOES, FINELY CHOPPED
- 4 SPRING ONIONS, FINELY SLICED
- SEEDS OF HALF A POMEGRANATE (OPTIONAL)

OMEGA DRESSING
SEE NEXT RECIPE

- FOR THE GARNISH
- HALF A HANDFUL OF FRESH DILL OR CHERVIL, FINELY CHOPPED (OPTIONAL)
- PUMPKIN SEEDS AND A HANDFUL OF WALNUTS, HAZELNUTS OR PISTACHIOS

METHOD

1. RINSE THE WILD RICE IN COLD WATER A FEW TIMES, PLACE IN A PAN AND COOK ACCORDING TO THE INSTRUCTIONS. THIS NORMALLY TAKES 45 TO 50 MINUTES DEPENDING ON THE VARIETY.
2. ONCE IT'S COOKED, DRAIN, FLUFF UP WITH A FORK AND ALLOW TO COOL.
3. MAKE THE DRESSING BY WHISKING ALL THE INGREDIENTS TOGETHER IN A SMALL BOWL OR JUST PUT THEM IN A GLASS JAR, PUT THE LID ON AND GIVE IT A GOOD SHAKE.
4. COMBINE THE REST OF THE INGREDIENTS IN A LARGE SALAD BOWL AND TOSS WELL TO MIX EVENLY, JUST USE YOUR HANDS, IT'S EASIER!
5. ADD THE DRESSING TO THE OTHER INGREDIENTS AND MIX WELL. YOU CAN USE HALF THE DRESSING FOR THIS SALAD AND KEEP THE REST IN THE FRIDGE IF YOU ARE BOTHERED ABOUT THE OIL.
6. GARNISH WITH PUMPKIN SEEDS AND CHOPPED NUTS. WALNUTS, HAZELNUTS AND PISTACHIOS ALL WORK WELL.

NOTES

RECIPE CARD

Omega dressing

A delicious dressing that is perfect with any salad or steamed veggies. Packed with health-giving ingredients & packs a real punch in the flavour department too!
This will make enough for a few salads. Store in the fridge and drizzle as needed

INGREDIENTS

- 6 TBSP EXTRA VIRGIN OLIVE OIL
- 2 TBSP BALSAMIC VINEGAR
- 1 SQUEEZE MAPLE SYRUP OR HONEY
- ½ TSP OF TURMERIC
- CLOVE OF GARLIC, CRUSHED
- SALT AND BLACK PEPPER

METHOD

JUST MEASURE ALL INGREDIENTS INTO A JAR, GIVE IT A GOOD SHAKE AND IT'S READY!

NOTES

RECIPE CARD

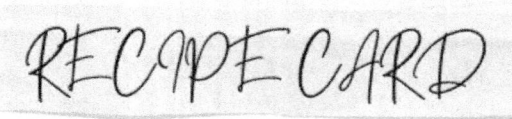

Fig and Olive Tapenade

INGREDIENTS

- 120G DRIED FIGS, ROUGHLY CHOPPED
- 120G BLACK KALAMATA OLIVES, PITTED
- 120G GREEN OLIVES, PITTED
- 3 TABLESPOONS EXTRA VIRGIN OLIVE OIL, PLUS EXTRA FOR THE TOP
- 1 TABLESPOON APPLE CIDER VINEGAR OR BALSAMIC VINEGAR
- 1 TEASPOON FRESH ROSEMARY, CHOPPED

METHOD

1. SIMPLY PUT ALL THE INGREDIENTS INTO A FOOD PROCESSOR OR BLENDER AND PULSE A FEW TIMES UNTIL YOU HAVE A ROUGH PASTE.
2. SPOON YOUR TAPENADE INTO A CLEAN GLASS JAR AND POUR A LITTLE OLIVE OIL OVER THE TOP TO PREVENT OXIDATION.
3. THIS WILL KEEP IN THE FRIDGE FOR UP TO TWO MONTHS.

NOTES

RECIPE CARD

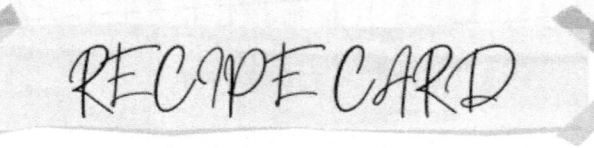

Beetroot & Walnut Dip

This is one of my favourite dips. It's just delicious and packed with health promoting ingredients! The addition of fermented garlic adds a healthy dose of probiotics, walnuts and extra virgin olive oil supply omega 3, tahini adds calcium and magnesium and beetroot contains nitrates which relax the blood vessels, reducing blood pressure and increasing blood flow to the brain!

This dip is great with raw veggies, on a baked sweet potato, in a wrap, sandwich or with oatcakes!

INGREDIENTS

- PACK OF VACUUM PACKED BEETROOT (250 TO 300G)
- ½ CUP WALNUTS
- 1 TABLESPOON TAHINI
- 1 TABLESPOON EXTRA VIRGIN OLIVE OIL
- 1 TABLESPOON BALSAMIC VINEGAR
- 1 CLOVE GARLIC OR FERMENTED GARLIC
- SEA SALT TO TASTE

METHOD

1. SIMPLY ADD ALL THE INGREDIENTS TO A BLENDER OR FOOD PROCESSOR AND BLITZ UNTIL BLENDED. A HAND HELD STICK BLENDER WORKS WELL TOO!
2. TRANSFER TO THE FRIDGE AND ENJOY!!

NOTES

RECIPE CARD

Pesto

Pesto is a fabulous way to up our intake of phytochemical rich herbs. It can be added to dips, sauces, pasta, or soups.
Any combination of greens can be used from kale, spinach, cavolo nero, wild garlic, basil, flat leaf parsley or coriander.
Any nuts or seeds, almonds, walnuts, pine nuts, brazil nuts, hazelnuts, pumpkin seeds or sunflower seeds.

INGREDIENTS

- 2 TIGHTLY PACKED CUPS OF GREENS
- 1 CUP OF MIXED NUTS AND SEEDS
- ½ CUP OLIVE OIL
- 1 TO 2 TABLESPOONS LEMON JUICE
- 1 OR 2 CLOVES CRUSHED GARLIC
- 1 TSP SEA SALT
- 1 TABLESPOON NUTRITIONAL YEAST FLAKES (OPTIONAL)

METHOD

1. SIMPLY ADD THE GREENS, NUTS, SEEDS, SALT, LEMON JUICE AND NUTRITIONAL YEAST TO A BLENDER. BLITZ A FEW TIMES THEN GRADUALLY ADD THE OIL WITH THE BLADE STILL RUNNING UNTIL FULLY COMBINED.
2. ADD EXTRA OIL IF YOU PREFER A THINNER CONSISTENCY.
3. STORE IN THE FRIDGE FOR 7 TO 10 DAYS.

NOTES

RECIPE CARD

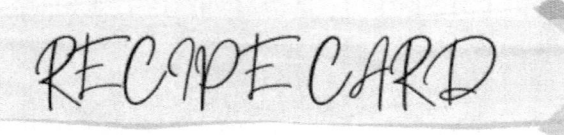

Tamari Toasted Seeds

A lovely crunchy addition to any meal, soup or salad or just enjoy a handful as a snack. Full of goodness too!

INGREDIENTS

- ½ CUP EACH OF
- SESAME
- SUNFLOWER
- PUMPKIN SEEDS
- 1 TEASPOON TAMARI
- SEAWEED FLAKES (OPTIONAL)

METHOD

1. HEAT A SMALL FRYING PAN AND TOAST SEEDS ON MEDIUM HEAT UNTIL LIGHTLY BROWN AND STARTING TO POP.
2. TURN OFF THE HEAT AND ADD TAMARI AND A SPRINKLING OF SEAWEED FLAKES.
3. MIX WELL THEN LEAVE TO COOL.
4. STORE IN AN AIRTIGHT CONTAINER.

NOTES

RECIPE CARD

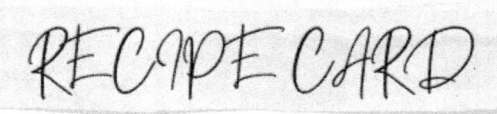

Beetroot Bliss Bites

These wee beetroot bites are delicious and just packed with prebiotics to nourish our gut microbes.

Makes 20 to 24

INGREDIENTS

- 100G TO 125G COOKED BEETROOT, APPROX 2 MEDIUM BEETS.
- 150G DATES, PRUNES OR FIGS
- 100G OATS
- 50G DESSICATED COCONUT
- 2 TBSP GROUND FLAXSEEDS
- 2 TBSP CHIA SEEDS
- 2 TBSP RAW CACAO
- 75G PUMPKIN SEEDS
- 75G SUNFLOWER SEEDS
- 3 TBSP COCONUT OIL

METHOD

1. SIMPLY BLITZ ALL THE INGREDIENTS IN A FOOD PROCESSOR UNTIL THEY COME TOGETHER.
2. TAKE SPOONFULS AND ROLL INTO BALLS.
3. SPRINKLE WITH RAW CACAO
4. STORE IN FRIDGE OR FREEZER

NOTES

RECIPE CARD

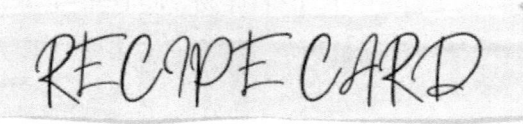

Probiotic Chocolate Bark

This is quite simply the most delicious thing ever!! I think I invented it, and boy it's a really great invention!

INGREDIENTS

- 2 BARS OF DARK CHOCOLATE (200G)
- TABLESPOON COCONUT OIL
- ¼ TO ½ CUP KEFIR OR A TABLESPOON OF TAHINI

TOPPING OPTIONS
- WEE SPRINKLING OF SEA SALT
- GOJI BERRIES
- SUNFLOWER SEEDS
- PUMPKIN SEEDS
- NUTS
- HEMP SEEDS
- COCONUT
- DRIED FRUIT

NOTES

METHOD

1. MELT 2 BARS OF DARK CHOCOLATE (200G) WITH A TABLESPOON COCONUT OIL. LET IT COOL A BIT, THEN ADD ¼ TO ½ CUP KEFIR OR A TABLESPOON OF TAHINI. MIX IT WELL THEN POUR ONTO A BAKING TRAY, LINED WITH GREASEPROOF PAPER.
2. POUR THE CHOCOLATE MIXTURE ONTO THE TRAY, SMOOTH IT OUT A BIT, THEN SPRINKLE LIBERALLY WITH TOPPINGS OF YOUR CHOICE! A WEE SPRINKLING OF SEA SALT IS A GREAT ADDITION, GOJI BERRIES, SUNFLOWER SEEDS, PUMPKIN SEEDS, NUTS, HEMP SEEDS, COCONUT, DRIED FRUIT ALL WORK WELL.
3. TRANSFER TO THE FREEZER AND FREEZE UNTIL SOLID THEN BREAK INTO PIECES AND ENJOY.
4. THIS IS BEST ENJOYED STRAIGHT FROM THE FREEZER!
5. YOU CAN UP THE ANTE ON THE HEALTH BENEFITS BY ADDING ½ TSP MACA, LUCUMA OR ANY SWEET SUPERFOOD POWDER WITH THE KEFIR.

RECIPE CARD

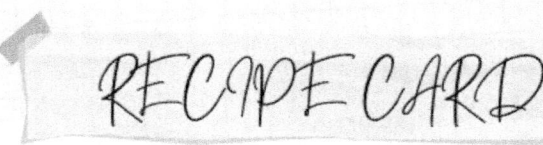

Radish Bombs

(Makes 1 litre jar)

I love these wee radishes, they are such a gorgeous colour and look great sliced in salads or added to stir fries at the last minute!

They are also a great digestive aid and will get your digestive juices flowing! The brine is a beautiful pink and can be used in salad dressings or just drink a small glass as a great tummy settler!

The brine is packed with probiotics!

INGREDIENTS

- 400G RADISHES, TOPS TRIMMED
- 1 OR 2 TSP PICKLING SPICE OR FENNEL OR CORIANDER OR FRESHLY GROUND BLACK PEPPER
- 15G/1 TABLESPOON SEA SALT
- 10G/2 TSP CASTER SUGAR
- 1 LITRE FILTERED WATER
- 1 RED ONION SLICED OR 5 SPRING ONIONS, WHITE BITS ONLY
- 3 SLICES FRESH GINGER
- 2 OR 3 LARGE SLICES OF LEMON
- 3 OR 4 GARLIC CLOVES, SMASHED WITH THE BACK OF A KNIFE
- 1 TSP OR MORE DRIED CHILLI FLAKES, DEPENDING HOW HOT YOU LIKE IT

METHOD

1. MAKE THE BRINE BY DISSOLVING THE SEA SALT AND SUGAR IN A JUG. WASH YOUR GLASS JAR IN HOT SOAPY WATER AND RINSE IT WELL TO REMOVE ANY SOAP RESIDUES.
2. PUT THE SPICES IN THE BOTTOM OF THE JAR, THEN ADD THE VEGETABLES, FINISHING WITH THE LEMON SLICES ON TOP. POUR THE BRINE OVER UNTIL EVERYTHING IS COMPLETELY SUBMERGED. COVER WITH A LARGE CABBAGE LEAF OR ZIPLOCK BAG FILLED WITH EXTRA BRINE TO KEEP EVERYTHING UNDER THE BRINE.
3. LOOSELY CLOSE THE JAR AND LEAVE SOMEWHERE COOL AND OUT OF DIRECT SUNLIGHT FOR 7 TO 12 DAYS.
4. TASTE THEM AFTER 7 DAYS AND IF THEY ARE SOUR ENOUGH FOR YOU THEN TRANSFER THEM TO THE FRIDGE WHERE THEY WILL KEEP FOR AROUND 6 MONTHS.
5. IF NOT SOUR ENOUGH THEN LEAVE THEM ANOTHER 4 OR 5 DAYS.
6. KEEP ANY EXCESS BRINE AND USE IT IN SALAD DRESSINGS, IT'S TEEMING WITH PROBIOTICS!!

NOTES

RECIPE CARD

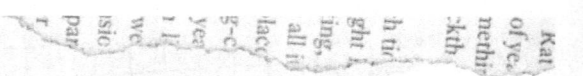

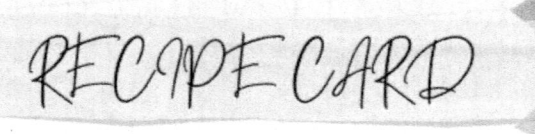

Fermented Indian Carrots

(These are a beautiful vibrant colour and packed with antiinflammatory ingredients. Perfect to accompany Indian food, tingle your taste buds and delight your gut microbes!
(Makes 1 litre jar)

INGREDIENTS

- 1 KG CARROTS, PEELED AND GRATED
- 1 KNOB FRESH GINGER, PEELED AND GRATED
- 2 TSP CHILLI FLAKES
- 2 TSP FENUGREEK
- 2 TSP MUSTARD SEED
- 1 TSP GROUND TURMERIC
- 20G SEA SALT AND FRESHLY GROUND BLACK PEPPER

METHOD

1. PLACE THE CARROTS IN A BOWL AND SPRINKLE WITH THE SEA SALT. SQUEEZE AND MASSAGE THE MIXTURE TO RELEASE SOME BRINE. THE CARROTS SHOULD START TO WILT AND BECOME WET.
2. ADD THE SPICES AND MIX TOGETHER USING A WOODEN SPOON, NOT YOUR HANDS OR THEY WILL BE STAINED ORANGE BY THE TURMERIC!
3. PACK THE MIXTURE INTO A CLEAN 1 LITRE GLASS JAR, PRESSING EACH HANDFUL DOWN FIRMLY TO ENSURE NO AIR IS TRAPPED. LEAVE 2.5CM HEADSPACE AT THE TOP OF THE JAR AND MAKE SURE THE CARROTS ARE COMPLETELY SUBMERGED UNDER THE BRINE.
4. CLOSE THE LID AND ALLOW TO FERMENT FOR 5 TO 7 DAYS AT ROOM TEMPERATURE.
5. STORE THE JAR IN THE FRIDGE AND USE WITHIN 6 MONTHS.

NOTES

RECIPE CARD

Switchel

Switchel is a great prebiotic drink, dating back to the Amish people. It's also called Haymakers Punch.
It contains some stellar ingredients, among them Apple Cider Vinegar, which is already naturally fermented, grated ginger, maple syrup and lemon juice.
Switchel restores electrolytes, eases pain and inflammation, balances Ph, keeps blood sugar levels balanced and aids digestion!
It's a very refreshing drink especially when diluted with sparkling water! Here is the simple recipe

INGREDIENTS

- 2 TABLESPOONS APPLE CIDER VINEGAR
- 3 TABLESPOONS MAPLE SYRUP
- 1 TABLESPOON GRATED GINGER
- 1 TABLESPOON LEMON JUICE
- 2 CUPS WATER
- 2 CUPS OF SPARKLING WATER TO SERVE

METHOD

1. SIMPLY ADD ALL THE INGREDIENTS TO A GLASS JAR, GIVE IT ALL A GOOD MIX, COVER AND THEN PUT IN THE FRIDGE OVERNIGHT.
2. TO SERVE, JUST MIX WITH AN EQUAL VOLUME OF SPARKLING WATER FOR A DELICIOUSLY REFRESHING DRINK!
3. ALTERNATIVELY, JUST ADD 4 CUPS OF WATER TO THE INGREDIENTS AT THE START AND SERVE AS IS! HAVING TRIED IT, IT'S DEFINITELY MORE REFRESHING WITH THE SPARKLING WATER BUT THAT'S JUST MY OPINION.
4. YOU CAN STRAIN THE GINGER OUT IF YOU DON'T FANCY LOTS OF BITS IN YOUR DRINK!

NOTES

Journal

For more movement and wellbeing support
Find Jen www.iamjenwilson.com

The Healing Rebel

Date:

MEALS:
BREAKFAST

LUNCH

DINNER

QUOTE OF THE DAY

MEDITATION

PRIORITIES
_____
_____
_____
_____

SELF-CARE
_____
_____
_____
_____

TO DO
_____
_____
_____
_____
_____
_____
_____
_____
_____
_____
_____
_____

WATER
○ ○ ○ ○
○ ○ ○ ○

3 WINS FROM YESTERDAY

GRATITUDE

The Healing Rebel

Date:

MEALS:
BREAKFAST

LUNCH

DINNER

QUOTE OF THE DAY

MEDITATION

PRIORITIES

SELF-CARE

TO DO

WATER
○ ○ ○ ○
○ ○ ○ ○

3 WINS FROM YESTERDAY

GRATITUDE

The Healing Rebel

Date:

MEALS:
BREAKFAST

LUNCH

DINNER

PRIORITIES
_____
_____
_____
_____

SELF-CARE
_____
_____
_____
_____

QUOTE OF THE DAY

TO DO
_____
_____
_____
_____
_____
_____
_____
_____
_____
_____
_____
_____

MEDITATION

WATER
○ ○ ○ ○
○ ○ ○ ○

3 WINS FROM YESTERDAY

GRATITUDE

The Healing Rebel

Date:

MEALS:
BREAKFAST

LUNCH

DINNER

QUOTE OF THE DAY

MEDITATION

PRIORITIES

SELF-CARE

TO DO

WATER
○ ○ ○ ○
○ ○ ○ ○

3 WINS FROM YESTERDAY

GRATITUDE

The Healing Rebel

Date:

MEALS:
BREAKFAST

LUNCH

DINNER

PRIORITIES

SELF-CARE

QUOTE OF THE DAY

TO DO

MEDITATION

WATER
○ ○ ○ ○
○ ○ ○ ○

3 WINS FROM YESTERDAY

GRATITUDE

The Healing Rebel

Date:

MEALS:
BREAKFAST

LUNCH

DINNER

PRIORITIES
_____
_____
_____
_____

SELF-CARE
_____
_____
_____
_____
_____

QUOTE OF THE DAY

TO DO
_____
_____
_____
_____
_____
_____
_____
_____
_____
_____
_____
_____
_____
_____

MEDITATION

WATER
○ ○ ○ ○
○ ○ ○ ○

3 WINS FROM YESTERDAY

GRATITUDE

The Healing Rebel

Date:

MEALS:
BREAKFAST

LUNCH

DINNER

QUOTE OF THE DAY

MEDITATION

PRIORITIES
_____
_____
_____
_____

SELF-CARE
_____
_____
_____
_____

TO DO
_____
_____
_____
_____
_____
_____
_____
_____
_____
_____
_____

WATER
○ ○ ○ ○
○ ○ ○ ○

3 WINS FROM YESTERDAY

GRATITUDE

The Healing Rebel

Date:

MEALS:
BREAKFAST

LUNCH

DINNER

QUOTE OF THE DAY

MEDITATION

PRIORITIES
_____
_____
_____
_____

SELF-CARE
_____
_____
_____
_____

TO DO
_____
_____
_____
_____
_____
_____
_____
_____
_____
_____
_____

WATER
○ ○ ○ ○
○ ○ ○ ○

3 WINS FROM YESTERDAY

GRATITUDE

The Healing Rebel

Date:

MEALS:

BREAKFAST

LUNCH

DINNER

QUOTE OF THE DAY

MEDITATION

PRIORITIES

SELF-CARE

TO DO

WATER
○ ○ ○ ○
○ ○ ○ ○

3 WINS FROM YESTERDAY

GRATITUDE

The Healing Rebel

Date:

MEALS:
BREAKFAST

LUNCH

DINNER

PRIORITIES
_____
_____
_____
_____

SELF-CARE
_____
_____
_____
_____
_____

TO DO
_____
_____
_____
_____
_____
_____
_____
_____
_____
_____
_____
_____
_____
_____

WATER
○ ○ ○ ○
○ ○ ○ ○

3 WINS FROM YESTERDAY

GRATITUDE

QUOTE OF THE DAY

MEDITATION

THE Healing REBEL

Date:

MEALS:
BREAKFAST

LUNCH

DINNER

QUOTE OF THE DAY

MEDITATION

PRIORITIES

SELF-CARE

TO DO

WATER
○ ○ ○ ○
○ ○ ○ ○

3 WINS FROM YESTERDAY

GRATITUDE

The Healing Rebel

Date:

MEALS:
BREAKFAST

LUNCH

DINNER

QUOTE OF THE DAY

MEDITATION

PRIORITIES
_____
_____
_____
_____

SELF-CARE
_____
_____
_____
_____
_____

TO DO
_____
_____
_____
_____
_____
_____
_____
_____
_____
_____
_____
_____
_____
_____

WATER
○ ○ ○ ○
○ ○ ○ ○

3 WINS FROM YESTERDAY

GRATITUDE

The Healing Rebel

Date:

MEALS:
BREAKFAST

LUNCH

DINNER

QUOTE OF THE DAY

MEDITATION

PRIORITIES

SELF-CARE

TO DO

WATER
○ ○ ○ ○
○ ○ ○ ○

3 WINS FROM YESTERDAY

GRATITUDE

The Healing Rebel

Date:

MEALS:
BREAKFAST

LUNCH

DINNER

QUOTE OF THE DAY

MEDITATION

PRIORITIES
_____
_____
_____
_____

SELF-CARE
_____
_____
_____
_____
_____

TO DO
_____
_____
_____
_____
_____
_____
_____
_____
_____
_____
_____
_____
_____

WATER
○ ○ ○ ○
○ ○ ○ ○

3 WINS FROM YESTERDAY

GRATITUDE

THE Healing REBEL

Date:

MEALS:
BREAKFAST

LUNCH

DINNER

QUOTE OF THE DAY

MEDITATION

PRIORITIES

SELF-CARE

TO DO

WATER
○ ○ ○ ○
○ ○ ○ ○

3 WINS FROM YESTERDAY

GRATITUDE

The Healing Rebel

Date:

MEALS:
BREAKFAST

LUNCH

DINNER

PRIORITIES
_____
_____
_____
_____

SELF-CARE
_____
_____
_____
_____
_____

QUOTE OF THE DAY

TO DO
_____
_____
_____
_____
_____
_____
_____
_____
_____
_____
_____
_____
_____

MEDITATION

WATER
○ ○ ○ ○
○ ○ ○ ○

3 WINS FROM YESTERDAY

GRATITUDE

The Healing Rebel

Date:

MEALS:
BREAKFAST

LUNCH

DINNER

QUOTE OF THE DAY

MEDITATION

PRIORITIES

SELF-CARE

TO DO

WATER
○ ○ ○ ○
○ ○ ○ ○

3 WINS FROM YESTERDAY

GRATITUDE

The Healing Rebel

Date:

MEALS:
BREAKFAST

LUNCH

DINNER

PRIORITIES
_____
_____
_____
_____

SELF-CARE
_____
_____
_____
_____
_____

QUOTE OF THE DAY

TO DO
_____
_____
_____
_____
_____
_____
_____
_____
_____
_____
_____
_____
_____
_____
_____

MEDITATION

WATER
○ ○ ○ ○
○ ○ ○ ○

3 WINS FROM YESTERDAY

GRATITUDE

The Healing Rebel

Date:

MEALS:
BREAKFAST

LUNCH

DINNER

PRIORITIES
_____
_____
_____
_____

SELF-CARE
_____
_____
_____
_____

QUOTE OF THE DAY

TO DO
_____
_____
_____
_____
_____
_____
_____
_____
_____
_____
_____
_____
_____
_____

MEDITATION

WATER
○ ○ ○ ○
○ ○ ○ ○

3 WINS FROM YESTERDAY

GRATITUDE

The Healing Rebel

Date:

MEALS:
BREAKFAST

LUNCH

DINNER

PRIORITIES
_____
_____
_____
_____

SELF-CARE
_____
_____
_____
_____

QUOTE OF THE DAY

TO DO
_____
_____
_____
_____
_____
_____
_____
_____
_____
_____
_____
_____

MEDITATION

WATER
○ ○ ○ ○
○ ○ ○ ○

3 WINS FROM YESTERDAY

GRATITUDE

The Healing Rebel

Date:

MEALS:
BREAKFAST

LUNCH

DINNER

PRIORITIES
_____
_____
_____

SELF-CARE
_____
_____
_____
_____

QUOTE OF THE DAY

TO DO
_____
_____
_____
_____
_____
_____
_____
_____
_____
_____
_____

MEDITATION

WATER
○ ○ ○ ○
○ ○ ○ ○

3 WINS FROM YESTERDAY

GRATITUDE

The Healing Rebel

Date:

MEALS:
BREAKFAST

LUNCH

DINNER

PRIORITIES
_____
_____
_____
_____

SELF-CARE
_____
_____
_____
_____

QUOTE OF THE DAY

TO DO
_____
_____
_____
_____
_____
_____
_____
_____
_____
_____
_____
_____

MEDITATION

WATER
○ ○ ○ ○
○ ○ ○ ○

3 WINS FROM YESTERDAY

GRATITUDE

The Healing Rebel

Date:

MEALS:
BREAKFAST

LUNCH

DINNER

PRIORITIES
_____
_____
_____
_____

SELF-CARE
_____
_____
_____
_____

WATER
○ ○ ○ ○
○ ○ ○ ○

3 WINS FROM YESTERDAY

QUOTE OF THE DAY

TO DO
_____
_____
_____
_____
_____

GRATITUDE

MEDITATION

The Healing Rebel

Date:

MEALS:
BREAKFAST

LUNCH

DINNER

PRIORITIES
_____
_____
_____
_____

SELF-CARE
_____
_____
_____
_____
_____

TO DO
_____
_____
_____
_____
_____
_____
_____
_____
_____
_____
_____
_____

WATER
○ ○ ○ ○
○ ○ ○ ○

3 WINS FROM YESTERDAY

GRATITUDE

QUOTE OF THE DAY

MEDITATION

The Healing Rebel

Date:

MEALS:
BREAKFAST

LUNCH

DINNER

PRIORITIES
_____
_____
_____
_____

SELF-CARE
_____
_____
_____
_____

QUOTE OF THE DAY

TO DO
_____
_____
_____
_____
_____
_____
_____
_____
_____
_____
_____
_____
_____

MEDITATION

WATER
○ ○ ○ ○
○ ○ ○ ○

3 WINS FROM YESTERDAY

GRATITUDE

The Healing Rebel

Date:

MEALS:
BREAKFAST

LUNCH

DINNER

PRIORITIES
_____
_____
_____
_____

SELF-CARE
_____
_____
_____
_____
_____

QUOTE OF THE DAY

TO DO
_____
_____
_____
_____
_____
_____
_____
_____
_____
_____
_____
_____
_____

MEDITATION

WATER
○ ○ ○ ○
○ ○ ○ ○

3 WINS FROM YESTERDAY

GRATITUDE

THE Healing REBEL

Date:

MEALS:
BREAKFAST

LUNCH

DINNER

PRIORITIES
_____
_____
_____
_____

SELF-CARE
_____
_____
_____
_____

QUOTE OF THE DAY

TO DO
_____
_____
_____
_____
_____
_____
_____
_____
_____
_____
_____
_____
_____

MEDITATION

WATER
○ ○ ○ ○
○ ○ ○ ○

3 WINS FROM YESTERDAY

GRATITUDE

The Healing Rebel

Date:

MEALS:
BREAKFAST

LUNCH

DINNER

QUOTE OF THE DAY

MEDITATION

PRIORITIES
_____
_____
_____

SELF-CARE
_____
_____
_____
_____

TO DO
_____
_____
_____
_____
_____
_____
_____
_____
_____
_____
_____

WATER
○ ○ ○ ○
○ ○ ○ ○

3 WINS FROM YESTERDAY

GRATITUDE

THE Healing REBEL

Date:

MEALS:
BREAKFAST

LUNCH

DINNER

PRIORITIES
_____
_____
_____

SELF-CARE
_____
_____
_____
_____

QUOTE OF THE DAY

TO DO
_____
_____
_____
_____
_____
_____

MEDITATION
_____
_____
_____
_____
_____

WATER
○ ○ ○ ○
○ ○ ○ ○

3 WINS FROM YESTERDAY

GRATITUDE

The Healing Rebel

Date:

MEALS:
BREAKFAST

LUNCH

DINNER

PRIORITIES
_____
_____
_____
_____

SELF-CARE
_____
_____
_____
_____

WATER
○ ○ ○ ○
○ ○ ○ ○

3 WINS FROM YESTERDAY

QUOTE OF THE DAY

TO DO
_____
_____
_____
_____
_____
_____
_____
_____
_____
_____
_____
_____
_____

GRATITUDE

MEDITATION

The Healing Rebel

Date:

MEALS:
BREAKFAST

LUNCH

DINNER

QUOTE OF THE DAY

MEDITATION

PRIORITIES
_____
_____
_____
_____

SELF-CARE
_____
_____
_____
_____

TO DO
_____
_____
_____
_____
_____
_____
_____
_____
_____
_____
_____
_____

WATER
○ ○ ○ ○
○ ○ ○ ○

3 WINS FROM YESTERDAY

GRATITUDE

The Healing Rebel

Date:

MEALS:
BREAKFAST

LUNCH

DINNER

QUOTE OF THE DAY

MEDITATION

PRIORITIES
_____
_____
_____
_____

SELF-CARE
_____
_____
_____
_____
_____

TO DO
_____
_____
_____
_____
_____
_____
_____
_____
_____
_____
_____
_____
_____
_____

WATER
○ ○ ○ ○
○ ○ ○ ○

3 WINS FROM YESTERDAY

GRATITUDE

The Healing Rebel

Date:

MEALS:
BREAKFAST

LUNCH

DINNER

PRIORITIES
_____
_____
_____
_____

SELF-CARE
_____
_____
_____
_____
_____
_____

QUOTE OF THE DAY

TO DO
_____
_____
_____
_____
_____
_____
_____
_____
_____
_____
_____

MEDITATION

WATER
○ ○ ○ ○
○ ○ ○ ○

3 WINS FROM YESTERDAY

GRATITUDE

THE Healing REBEL

Date:

MEALS:
BREAKFAST

LUNCH

DINNER

PRIORITIES

SELF-CARE

QUOTE OF THE DAY

TO DO

MEDITATION

WATER
○ ○ ○ ○
○ ○ ○ ○

3 WINS FROM YESTERDAY

GRATITUDE

The Healing Rebel

Date:

MEALS:
BREAKFAST

LUNCH

DINNER

PRIORITIES
_____
_____
_____

SELF-CARE
_____
_____
_____
_____

TO DO
_____
_____
_____
_____
_____
_____
_____
_____
_____
_____
_____
_____

WATER
○ ○ ○ ○
○ ○ ○ ○

3 WINS FROM YESTERDAY

GRATITUDE

QUOTE OF THE DAY

MEDITATION

The Healing Rebel

Date:

MEALS:
BREAKFAST

LUNCH

DINNER

PRIORITIES
_____
_____
_____

SELF-CARE
_____
_____
_____
_____

QUOTE OF THE DAY

TO DO
_____
_____
_____
_____
_____
_____
_____
_____
_____
_____
_____
_____

MEDITATION

WATER
○ ○ ○ ○
○ ○ ○ ○

3 WINS FROM YESTERDAY

GRATITUDE

The Healing Rebel

Date:

MEALS:
BREAKFAST

LUNCH

DINNER

PRIORITIES
_____
_____
_____

SELF-CARE
_____
_____
_____
_____

QUOTE OF THE DAY

TO DO
_____
_____
_____
_____
_____
_____
_____
_____
_____
_____
_____
_____

MEDITATION

WATER
○ ○ ○ ○
○ ○ ○ ○

3 WINS FROM YESTERDAY

GRATITUDE

The Healing Rebel

Date:

MEALS:
BREAKFAST

LUNCH

DINNER

PRIORITIES
_____
_____
_____

SELF-CARE
_____
_____
_____

QUOTE OF THE DAY

TO DO
_____
_____
_____
_____
_____
_____
_____
_____
_____
_____
_____
_____
_____

MEDITATION

WATER
○ ○ ○ ○
○ ○ ○ ○

3 WINS FROM YESTERDAY

GRATITUDE

THE Healing REBEL

Date:

MEALS:
BREAKFAST

LUNCH

DINNER

PRIORITIES
_____
_____
_____
_____

SELF-CARE
_____
_____
_____
_____

TO DO
_____
_____
_____
_____
_____
_____
_____
_____
_____
_____
_____
_____
_____

WATER
○ ○ ○ ○
○ ○ ○ ○

3 WINS FROM YESTERDAY

GRATITUDE

QUOTE OF THE DAY

MEDITATION

The Healing Rebel

Date:

MEALS:
BREAKFAST

LUNCH

DINNER

QUOTE OF THE DAY

MEDITATION

PRIORITIES
_____
_____
_____
_____

SELF-CARE
_____
_____
_____
_____

TO DO
_____
_____
_____
_____
_____
_____
_____
_____
_____
_____
_____
_____

WATER
○ ○ ○ ○
○ ○ ○ ○

3 WINS FROM YESTERDAY

GRATITUDE

The Healing Rebel

Date:

MEALS:
BREAKFAST

LUNCH

DINNER

PRIORITIES
_____
_____
_____
_____

SELF-CARE
_____
_____
_____
_____

TO DO
_____
_____
_____
_____
_____
_____
_____
_____
_____
_____
_____
_____
_____

QUOTE OF THE DAY

MEDITATION

WATER
○ ○ ○ ○
○ ○ ○ ○

3 WINS FROM YESTERDAY

GRATITUDE

The Healing Rebel

Date:

MEALS:
BREAKFAST

LUNCH

DINNER

QUOTE OF THE DAY

MEDITATION

PRIORITIES
_____
_____
_____

SELF-CARE
_____
_____
_____
_____

TO DO
_____
_____
_____
_____
_____
_____
_____
_____
_____
_____
_____
_____

WATER
○ ○ ○ ○
○ ○ ○ ○

3 WINS FROM YESTERDAY

GRATITUDE

The Healing Rebel

Date:

MEALS:
BREAKFAST

LUNCH

DINNER

PRIORITIES
_____
_____
_____
_____

SELF-CARE
_____
_____
_____
_____
_____

TO DO
_____
_____
_____
_____
_____
_____
_____
_____
_____
_____
_____
_____
_____
_____

QUOTE OF THE DAY

MEDITATION

WATER
○ ○ ○ ○
○ ○ ○ ○

3 WINS FROM YESTERDAY

GRATITUDE

The Healing Rebel

Date:

MEALS:
BREAKFAST

LUNCH

DINNER

QUOTE OF THE DAY

MEDITATION

PRIORITIES
_____
_____
_____

SELF-CARE
_____
_____
_____
_____
_____

TO DO
_____
_____
_____
_____
_____
_____
_____
_____
_____
_____
_____

WATER
○ ○ ○ ○
○ ○ ○ ○

3 WINS FROM YESTERDAY

GRATITUDE

The Healing Rebel

Date:

MEALS:
BREAKFAST

LUNCH

DINNER

QUOTE OF THE DAY

MEDITATION

PRIORITIES
_____
_____
_____
_____

SELF-CARE
_____
_____
_____
_____
_____

TO DO
_____
_____
_____
_____
_____
_____
_____
_____
_____
_____
_____
_____

WATER
○ ○ ○ ○
○ ○ ○ ○

3 WINS FROM YESTERDAY

GRATITUDE

The Healing Rebel

Date:

MEALS:
BREAKFAST

LUNCH

DINNER

QUOTE OF THE DAY

MEDITATION

PRIORITIES

SELF-CARE

TO DO

WATER
○ ○ ○ ○
○ ○ ○ ○

3 WINS FROM YESTERDAY

GRATITUDE

The Healing Rebel

Date:

MEALS:
BREAKFAST

LUNCH

DINNER

PRIORITIES
_____
_____
_____
_____

SELF-CARE
_____
_____
_____
_____

TO DO
_____
_____
_____
_____
_____
_____
_____
_____
_____
_____
_____
_____
_____

QUOTE OF THE DAY

MEDITATION

WATER
○ ○ ○ ○
○ ○ ○ ○

3 WINS FROM YESTERDAY

GRATITUDE

The Healing Rebel

Date:

MEALS:
BREAKFAST

LUNCH

DINNER

QUOTE OF THE DAY

MEDITATION

PRIORITIES
_____
_____
_____
_____

SELF-CARE
_____
_____
_____
_____

TO DO
_____
_____
_____
_____
_____
_____
_____
_____
_____
_____
_____
_____
_____

WATER
○ ○ ○ ○
○ ○ ○ ○

3 WINS FROM YESTERDAY

GRATITUDE

The Healing Rebel

Date:

MEALS:
BREAKFAST

LUNCH

DINNER

PRIORITIES
_____
_____
_____
_____

SELF-CARE
_____
_____
_____
_____

TO DO
_____
_____
_____
_____
_____
_____
_____
_____
_____
_____
_____

WATER
○ ○ ○ ○
○ ○ ○ ○

3 WINS FROM YESTERDAY

GRATITUDE

QUOTE OF THE DAY

MEDITATION

The Healing Rebel

Date:

MEALS:
BREAKFAST

LUNCH

DINNER

PRIORITIES
_____
_____
_____
_____

SELF-CARE
_____
_____
_____
_____

TO DO
_____
_____
_____
_____
_____
_____
_____
_____
_____
_____
_____
_____
_____

WATER
○ ○ ○ ○
○ ○ ○ ○

3 WINS FROM YESTERDAY

GRATITUDE

QUOTE OF THE DAY

MEDITATION

The Healing Rebel

Date:

MEALS:
BREAKFAST

LUNCH

DINNER

PRIORITIES
_____
_____
_____
_____

SELF-CARE
_____
_____
_____
_____

QUOTE OF THE DAY

TO DO
_____
_____
_____
_____
_____
_____
_____
_____
_____
_____

MEDITATION

WATER
○ ○ ○ ○
○ ○ ○ ○

3 WINS FROM YESTERDAY

GRATITUDE

The Healing Rebel

Date:

MEALS:
BREAKFAST

LUNCH

DINNER

QUOTE OF THE DAY

MEDITATION

PRIORITIES
_____
_____
_____

SELF-CARE
_____
_____
_____
_____

TO DO
_____
_____
_____
_____
_____
_____
_____
_____
_____
_____
_____
_____
_____

WATER
○ ○ ○ ○
○ ○ ○ ○

3 WINS FROM YESTERDAY

GRATITUDE

The Healing Rebel

Date:

MEALS:
BREAKFAST

LUNCH

DINNER

QUOTE OF THE DAY

MEDITATION

PRIORITIES
_____
_____
_____
_____

SELF-CARE
_____
_____
_____
_____

TO DO
_____
_____
_____
_____
_____
_____
_____
_____
_____
_____

WATER
○ ○ ○ ○
○ ○ ○ ○

3 WINS FROM YESTERDAY

GRATITUDE

The Healing Rebel

Date:

MEALS:
BREAKFAST

LUNCH

DINNER

PRIORITIES
_____
_____
_____

SELF-CARE
_____
_____
_____

QUOTE OF THE DAY

TO DO
_____
_____
_____
_____
_____
_____
_____
_____
_____
_____
_____
_____
_____
_____

MEDITATION

WATER
○ ○ ○ ○
○ ○ ○ ○

3 WINS FROM YESTERDAY

GRATITUDE

THE Healing REBEL

Date:

MEALS:
BREAKFAST

LUNCH

DINNER

QUOTE OF THE DAY

MEDITATION

PRIORITIES

SELF-CARE

TO DO

WATER
○ ○ ○ ○
○ ○ ○ ○

3 WINS FROM YESTERDAY

GRATITUDE

The Healing Rebel

Date:

MEALS:
BREAKFAST

LUNCH

DINNER

PRIORITIES
_____
_____
_____
_____

SELF-CARE
_____
_____
_____
_____
_____

TO DO
_____
_____
_____
_____
_____
_____
_____
_____
_____
_____
_____
_____
_____
_____

WATER
○ ○ ○ ○
○ ○ ○ ○

3 WINS FROM YESTERDAY

GRATITUDE

QUOTE OF THE DAY

MEDITATION

The Healing Rebel

Date:

MEALS:
BREAKFAST

LUNCH

DINNER

PRIORITIES

SELF-CARE

TO DO

WATER
○ ○ ○ ○
○ ○ ○ ○

3 WINS FROM YESTERDAY

QUOTE OF THE DAY

GRATITUDE

MEDITATION

The Healing Rebel

Date:

MEALS:
BREAKFAST

LUNCH

DINNER

QUOTE OF THE DAY

MEDITATION

PRIORITIES

SELF-CARE

TO DO

WATER
○ ○ ○ ○
○ ○ ○ ○

3 WINS FROM YESTERDAY

GRATITUDE

The Healing Rebel

Date:

MEALS:
BREAKFAST

LUNCH

DINNER

PRIORITIES
_____
_____
_____

SELF-CARE
_____
_____
_____
_____

TO DO
_____
_____
_____
_____
_____
_____
_____
_____
_____
_____
_____
_____

WATER
○ ○ ○ ○
○ ○ ○ ○

3 WINS FROM YESTERDAY

GRATITUDE

QUOTE OF THE DAY

MEDITATION

The Healing Rebel

Date:

MEALS:
BREAKFAST

LUNCH

DINNER

PRIORITIES
_____
_____
_____
_____

SELF-CARE
_____
_____
_____
_____

QUOTE OF THE DAY

TO DO
_____
_____
_____
_____
_____
_____
_____
_____
_____
_____
_____
_____

MEDITATION

WATER
○ ○ ○ ○
○ ○ ○ ○

3 WINS FROM YESTERDAY

GRATITUDE

The Healing Rebel

Date:

MEALS:
BREAKFAST

LUNCH

DINNER

PRIORITIES
_____
_____
_____
_____

SELF-CARE
_____
_____
_____
_____

QUOTE OF THE DAY

TO DO
_____
_____
_____
_____
_____
_____

MEDITATION
_____
_____
_____
_____

WATER
○ ○ ○ ○
○ ○ ○ ○

3 WINS FROM YESTERDAY

GRATITUDE

The Healing Rebel

Date:

MEALS:
BREAKFAST

LUNCH

DINNER

PRIORITIES
_____
_____
_____

SELF-CARE
_____
_____
_____
_____

QUOTE OF THE DAY

TO DO
_____
_____
_____
_____
_____
_____
_____
_____
_____
_____
_____
_____
_____

MEDITATION

WATER
○ ○ ○ ○
○ ○ ○ ○

3 WINS FROM YESTERDAY

GRATITUDE

The Healing Rebel

Date:

MEALS:
BREAKFAST

LUNCH

DINNER

QUOTE OF THE DAY

MEDITATION

PRIORITIES

SELF-CARE

TO DO

WATER
○ ○ ○ ○
○ ○ ○ ○

3 WINS FROM YESTERDAY

GRATITUDE

The Healing Rebel

Date:

MEALS:
BREAKFAST

LUNCH

DINNER

QUOTE OF THE DAY

MEDITATION

PRIORITIES
_____
_____
_____
_____

SELF-CARE
_____
_____
_____
_____

TO DO
_____
_____
_____
_____
_____
_____
_____
_____
_____
_____
_____

WATER
○ ○ ○ ○
○ ○ ○ ○

3 WINS FROM YESTERDAY

GRATITUDE

The Healing Rebel

Date:

MEALS:
BREAKFAST

LUNCH

DINNER

PRIORITIES
_____
_____
_____

SELF-CARE
_____
_____
_____
_____

TO DO
_____
_____
_____
_____
_____
_____
_____
_____
_____
_____

WATER
○ ○ ○ ○
○ ○ ○ ○

3 WINS FROM YESTERDAY

GRATITUDE

QUOTE OF THE DAY

MEDITATION

The Healing Rebel

Date:

MEALS:
BREAKFAST

LUNCH

DINNER

QUOTE OF THE DAY

MEDITATION

PRIORITIES
_____
_____
_____

SELF-CARE
_____
_____
_____
_____

TO DO
_____
_____
_____
_____
_____
_____
_____
_____
_____
_____
_____

WATER
○ ○ ○ ○
○ ○ ○ ○

3 WINS FROM YESTERDAY

GRATITUDE

The Healing Rebel

Date:

MEALS:
BREAKFAST

LUNCH

DINNER

PRIORITIES
_____
_____
_____

SELF-CARE
_____
_____
_____
_____

QUOTE OF THE DAY

TO DO
_____
_____
_____
_____
_____

MEDITATION
_____
_____
_____
_____
_____

WATER
○ ○ ○ ○
○ ○ ○ ○

3 WINS FROM YESTERDAY

GRATITUDE

THE Healing REBEL

Date:

MEALS:
BREAKFAST

LUNCH

DINNER

QUOTE OF THE DAY

MEDITATION

PRIORITIES
_____
_____
_____

SELF-CARE
_____
_____
_____
_____

TO DO
_____
_____
_____
_____
_____
_____
_____
_____
_____
_____
_____
_____

WATER
○ ○ ○ ○
○ ○ ○ ○

3 WINS FROM YESTERDAY

GRATITUDE

The Healing Rebel

Date:

MEALS:
BREAKFAST

LUNCH

DINNER

PRIORITIES
_____
_____
_____

SELF-CARE
_____
_____
_____
_____

QUOTE OF THE DAY

TO DO
_____
_____
_____
_____
_____
_____
_____
_____
_____
_____
_____
_____

MEDITATION

WATER
○ ○ ○ ○
○ ○ ○ ○

3 WINS FROM YESTERDAY

GRATITUDE

The Healing Rebel

Date:

MEALS:
BREAKFAST

LUNCH

DINNER

QUOTE OF THE DAY

MEDITATION

PRIORITIES

SELF-CARE

TO DO

WATER
○ ○ ○ ○
○ ○ ○ ○

3 WINS FROM YESTERDAY

GRATITUDE

THE Healing REBEL

Date:

MEALS:
BREAKFAST

LUNCH

DINNER

PRIORITIES
_____
_____
_____
_____

SELF-CARE
_____
_____
_____
_____
_____

TO DO
_____
_____
_____
_____
_____
_____
_____
_____
_____
_____
_____
_____

WATER
○ ○ ○ ○
○ ○ ○ ○

3 WINS FROM YESTERDAY

GRATITUDE

QUOTE OF THE DAY

MEDITATION

The Healing Rebel

Date:

MEALS:
BREAKFAST

LUNCH

DINNER

PRIORITIES
_____
_____
_____
_____

SELF-CARE
_____
_____
_____
_____

QUOTE OF THE DAY

TO DO
_____
_____
_____
_____
_____
_____
_____
_____

MEDITATION
_____
_____
_____
_____

WATER
○ ○ ○ ○
○ ○ ○ ○

3 WINS FROM YESTERDAY

GRATITUDE

The Healing Rebel

Date:

MEALS:
BREAKFAST

LUNCH

DINNER

PRIORITIES

SELF-CARE

QUOTE OF THE DAY

TO DO

MEDITATION

WATER
○ ○ ○ ○
○ ○ ○ ○

3 WINS FROM YESTERDAY

GRATITUDE

The Healing Rebel

Date:

MEALS:
BREAKFAST

LUNCH

DINNER

QUOTE OF THE DAY

MEDITATION

PRIORITIES

SELF-CARE

TO DO

WATER
○ ○ ○ ○
○ ○ ○ ○

3 WINS FROM YESTERDAY

GRATITUDE

The Healing Rebel

Date:

MEALS:
BREAKFAST

LUNCH

DINNER

PRIORITIES
_____
_____
_____
_____

SELF-CARE
_____
_____
_____
_____

TO DO
_____
_____
_____
_____
_____
_____
_____
_____
_____
_____
_____
_____
_____

WATER
○ ○ ○ ○
○ ○ ○ ○

3 WINS FROM YESTERDAY

GRATITUDE

QUOTE OF THE DAY

MEDITATION

The Healing Rebel

Date:

MEALS:
BREAKFAST

LUNCH

DINNER

QUOTE OF THE DAY

MEDITATION

PRIORITIES
_____
_____
_____
_____

SELF-CARE
_____
_____
_____
_____
_____

TO DO
_____
_____
_____
_____
_____
_____
_____
_____
_____
_____
_____
_____
_____

WATER
○ ○ ○ ○
○ ○ ○ ○

3 WINS FROM YESTERDAY

GRATITUDE

The Healing Rebel

Date:

MEALS:
BREAKFAST

LUNCH

DINNER

PRIORITIES
_____
_____
_____
_____

SELF-CARE
_____
_____
_____
_____
_____

TO DO
_____
_____
_____
_____
_____
_____
_____
_____
_____
_____
_____
_____
_____

QUOTE OF THE DAY

MEDITATION

WATER
○ ○ ○ ○
○ ○ ○ ○

3 WINS FROM YESTERDAY

GRATITUDE

The Healing Rebel

Date:

MEALS:
BREAKFAST

LUNCH

DINNER

PRIORITIES
_____
_____
_____
_____

SELF-CARE
_____
_____
_____
_____

QUOTE OF THE DAY

TO DO
_____
_____
_____
_____
_____
_____
_____
_____
_____
_____
_____
_____
_____
_____

MEDITATION

WATER
○ ○ ○ ○
○ ○ ○ ○

3 WINS FROM YESTERDAY

GRATITUDE

The Healing Rebel

Date:

MEALS:
BREAKFAST

LUNCH

DINNER

QUOTE OF THE DAY

MEDITATION

PRIORITIES
_____
_____
_____
_____

SELF-CARE
_____
_____
_____
_____

TO DO
_____
_____
_____
_____
_____
_____
_____
_____
_____
_____
_____
_____

WATER
○ ○ ○ ○
○ ○ ○ ○

3 WINS FROM YESTERDAY

GRATITUDE

The Healing Rebel

Date:

MEALS:
BREAKFAST

LUNCH

DINNER

QUOTE OF THE DAY

MEDITATION

PRIORITIES
_____
_____
_____
_____
_____

SELF-CARE
_____
_____
_____
_____
_____

TO DO
_____
_____
_____
_____
_____
_____
_____
_____
_____
_____
_____
_____
_____

WATER
○ ○ ○ ○
○ ○ ○ ○

3 WINS FROM YESTERDAY

GRATITUDE

The Healing Rebel

Date:

MEALS:
BREAKFAST

LUNCH

DINNER

PRIORITIES
_____
_____
_____
_____

SELF-CARE
_____
_____
_____
_____
_____

TO DO
_____
_____
_____
_____
_____
_____
_____
_____
_____
_____
_____

QUOTE OF THE DAY

MEDITATION

WATER
○ ○ ○ ○
○ ○ ○ ○

3 WINS FROM YESTERDAY

GRATITUDE

The Healing Rebel

Date:

MEALS:
BREAKFAST

LUNCH

DINNER

QUOTE OF THE DAY

MEDITATION

PRIORITIES
_____
_____
_____
_____

SELF-CARE
_____
_____
_____
_____

TO DO
_____
_____
_____
_____
_____
_____
_____
_____
_____
_____

WATER
○ ○ ○ ○
○ ○ ○ ○

3 WINS FROM YESTERDAY

GRATITUDE

The Healing Rebel

Date:

MEALS:
BREAKFAST

LUNCH

DINNER

PRIORITIES
_____
_____
_____
_____

SELF-CARE
_____
_____
_____
_____

TO DO
_____
_____
_____
_____
_____
_____
_____
_____
_____
_____
_____
_____

WATER
○ ○ ○ ○
○ ○ ○ ○

3 WINS FROM YESTERDAY

GRATITUDE

QUOTE OF THE DAY

MEDITATION

THE Healing REBEL

Date:

MEALS:
BREAKFAST

LUNCH

DINNER

PRIORITIES
_____
_____
_____

SELF-CARE
_____
_____
_____
_____

TO DO
_____
_____
_____
_____
_____
_____
_____
_____
_____
_____
_____
_____

WATER
○ ○ ○ ○
○ ○ ○ ○

3 WINS FROM YESTERDAY

GRATITUDE

QUOTE OF THE DAY

MEDITATION

The Healing Rebel

Date:

MEALS:
BREAKFAST

LUNCH

DINNER

PRIORITIES
_____
_____
_____
_____

SELF-CARE
_____
_____
_____
_____

QUOTE OF THE DAY

TO DO
_____
_____
_____
_____
_____
_____
_____
_____
_____
_____
_____
_____

MEDITATION

WATER
○ ○ ○ ○
○ ○ ○ ○

3 WINS FROM YESTERDAY

GRATITUDE

The Healing Rebel

Date:

MEALS:
BREAKFAST

LUNCH

DINNER

PRIORITIES
_____
_____
_____
_____

SELF-CARE
_____
_____
_____
_____

TO DO
_____
_____
_____
_____
_____
_____
_____
_____
_____
_____
_____
_____

WATER
○ ○ ○ ○
○ ○ ○ ○

3 WINS FROM YESTERDAY

GRATITUDE

QUOTE OF THE DAY

MEDITATION

The Healing Rebel

Date:

MEALS:
BREAKFAST

LUNCH

DINNER

PRIORITIES
_____
_____
_____
_____

SELF-CARE
_____
_____
_____
_____

TO DO
_____
_____
_____
_____
_____
_____
_____
_____
_____
_____
_____

WATER
○ ○ ○ ○
○ ○ ○ ○

3 WINS FROM YESTERDAY

GRATITUDE

QUOTE OF THE DAY

MEDITATION

THE Healing REBEL

Date:

MEALS:
BREAKFAST

LUNCH

DINNER

PRIORITIES
_____
_____
_____
_____

SELF-CARE
_____
_____
_____
_____

TO DO
_____
_____
_____
_____
_____
_____
_____
_____
_____
_____
_____
_____

WATER
○ ○ ○ ○
○ ○ ○ ○

3 WINS FROM YESTERDAY

GRATITUDE

QUOTE OF THE DAY

MEDITATION

The Healing Rebel

Date:

MEALS:
BREAKFAST

LUNCH

DINNER

PRIORITIES
_____
_____
_____
_____

SELF-CARE
_____
_____
_____
_____

QUOTE OF THE DAY

TO DO
_____
_____
_____
_____
_____
_____
_____
_____
_____
_____
_____
_____

MEDITATION

WATER
○ ○ ○ ○
○ ○ ○ ○

3 WINS FROM YESTERDAY

GRATITUDE

The Healing Rebel

Date:

MEALS:
BREAKFAST

LUNCH

DINNER

PRIORITIES
_____
_____
_____
_____

SELF-CARE
_____
_____
_____
_____

TO DO
_____
_____
_____
_____
_____
_____
_____
_____
_____
_____
_____
_____
_____

QUOTE OF THE DAY

MEDITATION

WATER
○ ○ ○ ○
○ ○ ○ ○

3 WINS FROM YESTERDAY

GRATITUDE

The Healing Rebel

Date:

MEALS:
BREAKFAST

LUNCH

DINNER

PRIORITIES
_____
_____
_____
_____

SELF-CARE
_____
_____
_____
_____

QUOTE OF THE DAY

TO DO
_____
_____
_____
_____
_____
_____
_____
_____
_____
_____
_____
_____

MEDITATION

WATER
○ ○ ○ ○
○ ○ ○ ○

3 WINS FROM YESTERDAY

GRATITUDE

THE Healing REBEL

Date:

MEALS:
BREAKFAST

LUNCH

DINNER

QUOTE OF THE DAY

MEDITATION

PRIORITIES

SELF-CARE

TO DO

WATER
○ ○ ○ ○
○ ○ ○ ○

3 WINS FROM YESTERDAY

GRATITUDE

The Healing Rebel

Date:

MEALS:
BREAKFAST

LUNCH

DINNER

PRIORITIES
_____
_____
_____

SELF-CARE
_____
_____
_____

TO DO
_____
_____
_____
_____
_____
_____
_____
_____
_____
_____

QUOTE OF THE DAY

MEDITATION

WATER
○ ○ ○ ○
○ ○ ○ ○

3 WINS FROM YESTERDAY

GRATITUDE

The Healing Rebel

Date:

MEALS:
BREAKFAST

LUNCH

DINNER

QUOTE OF THE DAY

MEDITATION

PRIORITIES
_____
_____
_____

SELF-CARE
_____
_____
_____
_____

TO DO
_____
_____
_____
_____
_____
_____
_____
_____
_____
_____

WATER
○ ○ ○ ○
○ ○ ○ ○

3 WINS FROM YESTERDAY

GRATITUDE

The Healing Rebel

Date:

MEALS:
BREAKFAST

LUNCH

DINNER

PRIORITIES
_____
_____
_____
_____

SELF-CARE
_____
_____
_____
_____
_____

TO DO
_____
_____
_____
_____
_____
_____
_____
_____
_____
_____
_____
_____

WATER
○ ○ ○ ○
○ ○ ○ ○

3 WINS FROM YESTERDAY

GRATITUDE

QUOTE OF THE DAY

MEDITATION

The Healing Rebel

Date:

MEALS:
BREAKFAST

LUNCH

DINNER

PRIORITIES
_____
_____
_____

SELF-CARE
_____
_____
_____
_____

QUOTE OF THE DAY

TO DO
_____
_____
_____
_____
_____
_____
_____
_____
_____
_____
_____
_____

MEDITATION

WATER
○ ○ ○ ○
○ ○ ○ ○

3 WINS FROM YESTERDAY

GRATITUDE

The Healing Rebel

Date:

MEALS:
BREAKFAST

LUNCH

DINNER

QUOTE OF THE DAY

MEDITATION

PRIORITIES

SELF-CARE

TO DO

WATER
○ ○ ○ ○
○ ○ ○ ○

3 WINS FROM YESTERDAY

GRATITUDE

The Healing Rebel

Date:

MEALS:
BREAKFAST

LUNCH

DINNER

QUOTE OF THE DAY

MEDITATION

PRIORITIES

SELF-CARE

TO DO

WATER
○ ○ ○ ○
○ ○ ○ ○

3 WINS FROM YESTERDAY

GRATITUDE

The Healing Rebel

Date:

MEALS:
BREAKFAST

LUNCH

DINNER

PRIORITIES
_____
_____
_____
_____

SELF-CARE
_____
_____
_____
_____
_____

QUOTE OF THE DAY

TO DO
_____
_____
_____
_____
_____
_____
_____

MEDITATION
_____
_____
_____
_____
_____

WATER
○ ○ ○ ○
○ ○ ○ ○

3 WINS FROM YESTERDAY

GRATITUDE

The Healing Rebel

Date:

MEALS:
BREAKFAST

LUNCH

DINNER

QUOTE OF THE DAY

MEDITATION

PRIORITIES
_____
_____
_____
_____

SELF-CARE
_____
_____
_____
_____
_____

TO DO
_____
_____
_____
_____
_____
_____
_____
_____
_____
_____
_____
_____

WATER
○ ○ ○ ○
○ ○ ○ ○

3 WINS FROM YESTERDAY

GRATITUDE

The Healing Rebel

Date:

MEALS:
BREAKFAST

LUNCH

DINNER

PRIORITIES
_____
_____
_____
_____

SELF-CARE
_____
_____
_____
_____

QUOTE OF THE DAY

TO DO
_____
_____
_____
_____
_____
_____
_____

MEDITATION
_____
_____
_____
_____
_____

WATER
○ ○ ○ ○
○ ○ ○ ○

3 WINS FROM YESTERDAY

GRATITUDE

THANK YOU

We hope you have loved using the recipes & journal. If you would like to buy yourself a new journal or gift one to a friend or family member, just head over to Amazon and search The Healing Rebel, Nourished By Nature Recipes & Journal

You will be continuing to support small businesses in Glasgow

Find Jen www.iamjenwilson.com
Find Janice www.blognourishedbynature.com

Printed in Great Britain
by Amazon